Bariatric Cookbook

Delicious Recipes for Your Gastric Sleeve Recovery

Table of Contents

Introduction

Congratulations on downloading the *Bariatric Cookbook: Delicious Recipes for Your Gastric Sleeve Recovery*. Thank you for doing so.

This is a must for your personal library. The *Bariatric Cookbook: Delicious Recipes for Your Gastric Sleeve Recovery* will provide you with many new dishes you never thought would be possible to prepare and remain healthy.

You will soon discover within the pages of this cookbook that you are truly entering a new stage of your life. You have the tools to continue down the right path to a much healthier future.

These are just a few of the recipes you can enjoy:

- Carrot Ginger Muffins
- Grilled Honey Garlic Pork Chops
- Chicken Enchiladas and Sour Cream
- Sunshine Fruit Salad
- Vegetarian Philly Cheese steak Sandwich
- Chili Popcorn
- Cinnamon Almond Raisins Snack

So many more!

The following chapters will discuss many variations of how you can improve your current lifestyle by changing the ways to prepare your meals. Each section is divided into breakfast, lunch, dinner, and snacks including something for the sweeter versions you always have a craving for when you are changing your eating patterns.

There are plenty of books on this subject on the market, thanks again for choosing this one! Every effort was made to ensure it is full of as much useful information as possible. Please enjoy!

Happy Cooking!

Chapter 1: Breakfast

Many of the recipes provided in this informative cookbook require you testing for doneness. This can be done by poking the cake/muffin or other product with a toothpick in the center. If it comes out clean – it's done.

Several abbreviations are also used in the nutrition counts:
- Calories: Cal
- Protein: P
- Carbs: C
- Fat: F

Baked Egg Cups

Ingredients
6 eggs
6 slices deli ham – lean
½ cup 2% cheddar cheese – shredded
1 tablespoon chopped chives
Pepper
Non-stick cooking spray

Instructions
1. Set the oven temperature at 350°F.
2. Lightly spray 6 muffin tins and arrange the ham slices to line the cups.
3. Bake ten minutes. Take the pan out and an egg to each cup.
4. Break the yolk and add a sprinkle of pepper.
5. Bake another 10 minutes if they are done to your preference. Garnish with cheese and chives.

Yields: Six servings
Cal: 125.6| P: 14.1 g | C: 0.9 g | F: 6.9 g

Crustless Quiche

Ingredients
2 cups egg beaters/egg whites
1 cup cottage cheese (non-fat)
½ cup each:
- Chopped – cooked broccoli
- Diced lean ham
- Colby or cheddar shredded cheese

Cooking spray
Pepper and salt to taste

Instructions
1. Set the oven temperature to 375°F. Spray a casserole dish with the cooking spray.
2. Blend all of the fixings and empty into the prepared casserole dish.
3. Bake 45 minutes until the center is set.

Yields: Six servings
Cal: 106.8| P: 18.7 g | C: 4.5 g | F: 1.4 g

Eggs and Oats

Ingredients
2 egg whites
1 whole egg
2 ounces skim milk
½ cup rolled oats (Quaker)
Optional Garnishes:
- Hot sauce
- Cayenne
- Honey cinnamon berries

Instructions

1. Use some non-stick cooking spray to lightly grease a skillet. Add all of the ingredients.
2. Cook as with any scrambled egg.

Yields: One serving
Cal: 272.6 | P: 20.2 g | C: 30.2 g | F: 8.0g

Egg in a Basket

Ingredients
1 large egg
1 slice of bread
Butter flavored cooking spray

Instructions
1. Remove the middle out of the slice of bread using a glass.
2. Use some cooking spray on a griddle with the medium heat setting.
3. Arrange the bread on the skillet/griddle and add the broken egg.
4. Cook until done.

Yields: One serving
Cal: 246.2 | P: 18.2 g | F: 10 g | C: 22.8 g

Light French Toast

Ingredients
¼ cup non-fat milk
2 slices whole wheat bread
½ cup egg beaters
1 teaspoon each:
- Splenda
- Vanilla extract
- Cinnamon

Instructions

1. Spray a frying pan with some non-stick cooking oil using medium-low heat.
2. Mix all of the components together except the bread.
3. Dip all sides of the bread into the mixture and cook three to four minutes per side.
4. Garnish with your favorite toppings (adding the calories).

Yields: One serving
Cal: 179.6 | P: 20.4 g | C: 26 g | F: 1.1 g

Sausage and Mushroom Gravy

Ingredients
8 ounces/2 cups chopped mushrooms**
¼ large chopped onions
2 tablespoons each:
- Olive oil
- Whole wheat flour

¼ teaspoon each:
- Black pepper
- Red pepper flakes
- Dried sage

½ teaspoon dried thyme
1 ½ cups skim milk

Instructions

1. Pour the oil and add the onions into a sauté pan. After two minutes, toss in the mushrooms and continue cooking another three to four minutes.
2. Add the flour, stirring for one minute, and add the spices.
3. Gently, add the milk, stirring until it's creamy. Simmer about five more minutes.
   **For best results use white button or baby bella mushrooms.

Yields: Four servings
Cal: 115.4 | P: 4.9 g | C: 9.4 g | F: 7 g

Sausage, Egg, and Cheese Roll-Ups

Ingredients
2 sliced mushrooms
½ cup egg substitute
2 tablespoons red onion
¼ cup each bell pepper:
  - Red
  - Green
2 turkey sausages (precooked)
½ cup torn spinach
2 tortillas (whole wheat)
¼ cup shredded cheddar cheese

Instructions
1. Ahead of time, prepare the sausage and chop the onions and peppers.
2. Prepare the skillet with the non-stick spray and scramble the egg with the veggies and sausage. Add the cheese and let it melt.
3. Arrange the tortillas on top of the eggs to warm for a few seconds.
4. Fill the tortillas with the ingredients, roll, and serve.

Yields: Two servings
Cal: 220.9 | P: 19.9 g | C: 19.3 g | F: 10.7 g

Spinach and Feta Egg Whites

Ingredients
2 cups baby spinach
3 egg whites

1 chopped tomato
¼ cup each:
- Chopped onion
- Crumbled feta cheese

Instructions
1. Chop the veggies and add them in a pan using medium heat, cooking the onions until they are translucent.
2. Add the spinach, tomato, and egg whites.
3. Before removing the pan from the burner, add ½ of the cheese to the mixture.
4. Top it off with the remainder of cheese, pepper, and salt.

Yields: One serving
Cal: 200.3 | P: 18.4 g | C: 13.0 g | F: 8.7 g

Muffins

Blueberry Muffin

Ingredients
½ tsp. salt
1 cup each:
- Flour
- Old-fashioned oats

1 tsp. each:
- Cinnamon
- Baking soda

½ cup each:
- Unsweetened applesauce
- Water
- Sugar

2 egg whites
1 cup frozen blueberries

Instructions

1. Prepare 12 muffin tins and program the oven to 350°F.
2. Combine the salt, soda, cinnamon, oats, and flour.
3. Add the egg whites, sugar, water, and apple sauce.
4. Blend in the blueberries.
5. Bake twenty to twenty-five minutes.

Yields: 12 servings
Cal: 102.8 | P: 3 g | C: 22 g | F: 0.9 g

Carrot Ginger Muffins

Ingredients
2 tablespoons butter
1 ½ teaspoons baking powder
1 cup flour (whole wheat)
1/3 cup each:

- White sugar
- Brown sugar

1 large finely shredded carrot
¼ cup skim milk
1 beaten egg
1 teaspoon fresh ginger (minced or shredded)
1/8 teaspoon each:

- Dry powdered ginger
- Cinnamon
- Allspice

1/8 tablespoon vanilla
Optional: ½ cut nuts/raisins (not in the counts)

Instructions

1. Program the oven temperature to 350°F.
2. Dice up the butter to soften in small cubes.
3. Combine the baking powder, flour, and butter - making fine pieces.

4. Add the ginger, sugars, milk, carrot, beaten egg, spices, and vanilla in a mixing container. Blend in the nuts and raisins (if using).
5. Add to 12 papered/lightly greased muffin tins.
6. Bake 25 minutes.

Yields: 12 servings
Cal: 99.6 | P: 2 g | C: 19.9 g | F: 2.5 g

Pumpkin Muffins

Ingredients
1 can (1 pound) pumpkin
1 box spice cake mix
½ cup flaxseed meal

Instructions
1. Program the oven to 350°F.
2. Add paper liners to a muffin tin or use cooking spray.
3. Combine all of the ingredients and bake 25 minutes.
4. Test with a toothpick for doneness.

Yields: 18 servings
Cal: 340 | P: 6 g | C: 53.0g | F: 12.5 g

Wheat, Bran, and Flaxseed Muffins

Ingredients
1 cup each:
- Oat bran
- Whole wheat flour
- Brown sugar
- Ground flaxseed

2 tsp. baking soda
2 tbsp. cinnamon
1 tsp. baking powder

2-3 apples
1 ½ - cups shredded carrots
¾ cup 2% milk
2 beaten eggs
½ tsp. salt
1 tsp. vanilla
½ cup each (*Optional*):
- Raisins
- Chopped nuts

Instructions
1. Prepare 24 paper liners/oil lined muffin tin. Set the oven to 350°F.
2. Core and chop the apples.
3. Blend the sugar, bran, flaxseed, flour, and other dry ingredients.
4. Shred the apples and carrots and toss with the nuts and raisins and all dry ingredients.
5. Whip the eggs, milk, and vanilla. Blend into the dry mixture.
6. Fill each cup ¾ full. Bake for 2- to 25 minutes.

Yields: 24 servings
Cal: 115.7 | P: 2.9 g | C: 20.8 g | F: 3.4 g

Zucchini Bread Muffins

Ingredients
3 large egg whites
1 tbsp. vanilla
2 cups of each:
- White sugar
- Grated zucchini
1 cup applesauce
1 tsp. baking soda

½ tsp. salt

3 cups flour (whole wheat)

2 tsp. each:

- Cinnamon
- Baking powder

3 tsp. brown sugar

Instructions
1. Set the oven temperature to 350°F.
2. Grease 24 muffin tins with some non-stick cooking spray.
3. Combine the sugar and eggs along with the applesauce, vanilla, and zucchini.
4. Slowly, blend in the dry components and b lend well.
5. Pour the batter and sprinkle each one with a pinch of brown sugar.
6. Bake twenty or thirty minutes or perform the toothpick test for doneness.

Yields: 24 servings

Cal: 139.6 | P: 3 g | C: 31.3 g | F: 0.9 g

Oats

Apple Cinnamon Oatmeal – Slow Cooker

Ingredients

2 Granny smith apples

1 teaspoon cinnamon

2 cups rolled oats

½ cup 2% evaporated milk

6 cups water

Instructions
1. Peel and dice the apples.

2. Spray the inside of the slow cooker with a bit of cooking spray.
3. Empty all of the fixings into the pot and add the water.
4. Place the lid on the cooker for eight to nine hours (low).

Yields: Six servings – one cup each
Cal: 167.8 | P: 5.7 g | C: 30.7 g | F: 3 g

Blue Oatmeal

Ingredients
2 tablespoons flaxseed (ground flax)
1 cup 100% natural whole grain oatmeal
2 teaspoons brown sugar
1 ½ - cups water
½ tablespoon unsweetened dry cocoa powder
½ cup frozen - unsweetened blueberries

Instructions
1. Add the dry ingredients to boiling water in a pan.
2. Reduce the heat and continue cooking two to three minutes on low heat.
3. Stir in the frozen berries and enjoy.

Yields: Two servings
Cal: 214.2 | P: 6.9 g | C: 38.4 g | F: 5.7 g

Pumpkin Pie Oatmeal

Ingredients
½ cup each:
- Uncooked old-fashioned oatmeal
- Canned pumpkin

Pinch of ground cardamom
1 cup non-fat milk

1 tablespoon sugar
¼ teaspoon pumpkin pie spice

Instructions
1. Combine all of the components and heat on low for 20 minutes until thick.

Yields: Two servings
Cal: 164.2 | P: 7.4 g | C: 30.9 g | F: 1.9 g

Summertime Uncooked Oatmeal

Ingredients
About 25 raisins
½ cup each:
- Milk
- Oats

1 teaspoon cinnamon

Instructions
1. Mix the ingredients in a tightly closed container and put them in the fridge overnight to blend.
2. Enjoy a healthy breakfast in the next morning without any cooking.

Yields: One serving
Cal: 391.3 | P: 17.9 g | C: 69.8 g | F: 5.7 g

Pancakes

Banana Bread Pancakes

Ingredients
2 pouches Quaker Instant Oatmeal – Banana Bread – weight control

2/3 cup cottage cheese

2 eggs or ½ cup egg beaters

Garnish: Cinnamon and vanilla extract

Instructions
1. Combine all of the components for the pancakes into a blender.
2. Cook over med-high setting on the stovetop.
3. Make 8 (6 inch) pancakes and enjoy.

Yields: Four servings

Cal: 126.2 | P: 10.7 g | C: 17.7 g| F: 1.5 g

Cheesecake Pancakes

Ingredients

4 ounces cream cheese

2 large eggs

Splenda to taste

1 tablespoon flaxseed

½ teaspoon ground cinnamon

Instructions
1. Use a mixer to whip the egg whites into stiff peaks.
2. Drop the cheese into a mixing container and blend with the mixer until smooth. Combine this with the yolks and sweetener, flaxseed meal, salt, and cinnamon. Fold in the whipped eggs.
3. Using med-low heat, lightly grease a fry pan.
4. Use ¼ cup per pancake and cook for two to three minutes per side.

Yields: Two servings

Cal: 293.5 | P: 11.1 g | C: 2.1 g | F: 26.4 g

Cinnamon Pancakes

Ingredients
1 ¼ - cup whole wheat flour
1 tsp. baking soda
2 tbsp. each:
- Cinnamon
- Splenda

½ cup egg beaters
1 cup skim milk
1 tbsp. vanilla extract

Instructions
1. Combine the Splenda, flour, and soda in a mixing dish.
2. Blend the vanilla, milk, and eggs. Slowly, add in the dry ingredients (step 1). Add the cinnamon last.
3. Pour the batter into the pan 1/3 cup for each pancake.

Yields: Eight servings
Cal: 92.6 | P: 5.1 g | C: 18.1 g | F: 0.4 g

Cottage Cheese and Oatmeal Pancakes

Ingredients
4 egg whites
1-2 packets Stevia
½ cup each:
- Dry oatmeal
- Fat-free cottage cheese

½ teaspoon each:
- Vanilla
- Baking powder

Instructions

1. Add all of the fixings, except for the oats and blend until smooth.
   Add the oats a little at a time.
2. Toss in berries if you like, but add them after the mixture is blended.
3. Cook the pancakes until done and top with your favorite sugar-free syrup.

Yields: Six servings
Cal: 47.5 | P: 5.8 g | C: 4.6 g | F: 0.5 g

Oatmeal Pancakes

Ingredients
1 large egg
1 tsp. baking powder
1 cup flour - whole wheat
1 ¼ cup each:
  - Old Fashioned Quaker Oats
  - Skim milk
1 tbsp. light olive oil

Instructions

1. Combine the milk and oats in a mixing dish and let them set for five minutes.
2. Pour the oil and egg in, and mix with the dry ingredients.
3. Add the batter ¼ of a cup at a time into a lightly greased skillet. Cook until browned. Flip over and cook until done.
4. Top it off with some yogurt, maple syrup, preserves or others (not counted in nutritional counts).

Yields: Four servings
Cal: 271.3 | P: 11.3 g | C: 43.1 g | F: 7.0 g

Cold Breakfast Treats

Chocolate Covered Strawberries Smoothie

Ingredients
1 cup milk (fat-free)
½ cup frozen strawberries
1 package instant breakfast/chocolate flavor (1/4 cup)
6 ounces strawberry yogurt

Instructions
1. Mix all of the components in the recipe using a processor or blender.
2. Puree for 1 minute.
3. *Note*: I used Carnation Breakfast.

Yields: Two servings
Cal: 140.9 | P: 9.3 g | C: 23.8 g | F: 0.5 g

Going Green Smoothie

Ingredients
1 medium banana
7 large strawberries
Up to:
- 2 ½ cups spinach leaves
- ¾ cup orange juice

Instructions
1. Add each of the fixings into the blender. Add some ice and enjoy.

Yields: Two cups - One serving
Cal: 233.9 | P: 5.2 g | C: 55.9 g | F: 1.4 g

Mixed Berry Smoothie

Ingredients
1 cup of each:
- Skim milk
- Fat-free yogurt

¾ cup frozen assorted berries/your choice
Optional: ¼ cup sugar

Instructions
1. Empty the yogurt and milk into a blender along with the berries.
2. Add some protein powder if you choose and enjoy.

Yields: Two servings
Cal: 257.8| P: 11.1 g | C: 47.4 g | F: 2.8 g

Peanut Butter Banana Smoothie

Ingredients
1 medium banana
1 cup non-fat milk
2 tbsp. peanut butter

Instructions
1. Combine everything in the blender with ice. Blend until creamy.

Yields: One serving
Cal: 374.3 | P: 17.6 g | C: 53.5 g | F: 12 g

Pumpkin Smoothie

Ingredients
1 cup ice cubes
½ of banana

1 teaspoon pumpkin spice
1 container (6 ounces) fat-free vanilla Greek yogurt
½ cup canned pumpkin

Instructions
Combine all of the goodies into the processor or blender. Puree until creamy.

Yields: One serving
Cal: 235.8 | P: 18 g | C: 40.7 g | F: 0.6 g

Strawberry Banana Smoothie

Ingredients
¾ cup non-fat milk
1cup frozen strawberries – unsweetened
2 small bananas – in chunks
1 container (8 ounces) strawberry-banana yogurt (low-fat)

Instructions
1. Blend the bananas frozen berries, milk, and yogurt.
2. Mix until smooth and serve.

Yields: Two servings
Cal: 261.2 | P: 8.5 g | C: 55.9g | F: 2 g

Yogurt Breakfast Popsicles

Ingredients
1 cup of each:
  - Chopped fruits/mixed berries
  - Non-fat plain Greek yogurt
½ cup each:
  - Instant/regular oats
  - Skim/1% milk

Also Needed: Popsicle molds

Instructions
1. Combine the yogurt and milk and pour into two molds.
2. Add a few berries to each one along with half of the oatmeal.
3. Add an ice cream stick to each mold and freeze for a minimum of four hours.

Yields: Six servings
Cal: 75 | P: 5 g | C: 11 g | F: 0.6 g

Chapter 2: Lunch: Salads and Pasta Dishes

Caprese Salad

Ingredients
6 ounces strawberries
1 ripe avocado
1 (7 ounces) sliced mozzarella ball
Small handful salad leaves
2-3 tablespoons balsamic dressing – your choice
Pepper and salt

Instructions
1. Toss in the salad leaves, avocado, strawberries, and cheese into a serving dish.
2. Drizzle with the dressing, salt, and pepper. Gently toss.

Yields: Two servings
Cal: 375| P: 23.8g | C: 13 g| F: 24.6 g

California Roll in a Bowl

Ingredients
1 head chopped lettuce
1 cup cooked brown rice
1 English cucumber – seedless – thinly sliced
1 (8 ounces) package cooked shrimp/crabmeat – chopped
1 grated carrot
1 ripe diced avocado
3 tablespoons pickled ginger

Ingredients for the Dressing
1 tablespoon light soy sauce

½ teaspoon wasabi powder – to taste
3 tablespoons rice wine vinegar

Garnishes:
1 large sheet seaweed/nori (toasted and in small bits)
1 tablespoon sesame seeds

Instructions
1. Combine all of the fixings for the dressing in a dish and whisk well.
2. Put the salad together by mixing and dividing all components into four sections.

Note: You can locate the ginger in the Asian section of the supermarket.

Yields: Four servings
Cal: 199.1 | P: 6.5 g | C: 27.3 g | F: 8.3 g

Caramel Apple Salad

Ingredients
1 tub (8 ounces) Cool Whip Free
1 can (14 ounces) pineapple tidbits with the juice
1 box instant butter scotch pudding mix (sugar-free)
4 large each:
- Fuji apples/Red Delicious
- Granny Smith apples

Instructions
1. Mix the pineapple with its juice and the pudding mix in a large mixing container.
2. Dice the apples into small bits and combine with the mixture.
3. Fold in the Cool Whip, mix well, and chill.

Yields: 16 servings
Cal: 90.7 | P: 0.2 g | C: 20.1 g | F: 0.4 g

Chickpea and Feta Salad

Ingredients
¾ cup chopped raw vegetables
2 tbsp. olive oil
¼ cup each:
- Can/fresh chickpeas
- Feta cheese

1 tsp. dried oregano
1 tbsp. lemon juice
Dash each of:
- Pepper
- Salt

Instructions
1. Crumble the feta cheese.
2. You can use your imagination for the chopped veggies. Include peppers, avocado, tomatoes, onions, and celery or your favorites.
3. Rinse and drain the chickpeas.
4. Combine all of the ingredients and leave the salad in the refrigerator until you are ready to eat.

Yields: One serving
Cal: 285.2 | P: 10.2 g | C: 22.2 g | F: 18.4 g

Coleslaw

Ingredients
1 small shredded carrot
3 cups green cabbage – shredded
¼ cup minced onion

1 tablespoon vinegar

1/3 cup mayonnaise

2 teaspoons sugar

½ teaspoon each:
- Celery seed
- Salt

Instructions
1. Prepare the onion, carrots, and cabbage into a bowl.
2. Blend the dressing well and dump it over the slaw.

Yields: Six servings

Cal: 71.7 | P: 0.8 g | C: 7.9 g | F: 4.5 g

Cucumber and Onion Salad with Vinegar

Ingredients

Pinch of salt and pepper

1 red onion

3-5 cucumbers (peeled)

½ cup each:
- White vinegar
- Water

1/3 cup sugar

Instructions
1. Slice the cucumbers and onions very thin and add to a salad dish.
2. Combine the water, vinegar, salt, pepper, and sugar and pour over the veggies.
3. Add a cover and marinate for a minimum of one hour.

Yields: Six servings

Cal: 67.5 | P: 1.3 g | C: 16.9 g | F: 0.2 g

Egg Salad

Ingredients
3 celery stalks
2 tablespoons pickle relish
6 large hard-boiled eggs
¼ cup of each:
- Diced onions
- Reduced fat mayonnaise

Optional:
- Pepper
- 1 teaspoon mustard

Dash of each:
- Celery seed
- Paprika

Instructions
1. Peel and chop the eggs, celery, and onions.
2. Combine all of the fixings and cover in the refrigerator until ready for your meal.

Yields: Six servings
Cal: 115.7 | P: 6.6 g | C: 4.3 g | F: 7.7 g

Grape Salad

Ingredients
2-4 pounds of grapes (green, red, or both)
1 package of fat-free– 8 ounces each:
- Sour cream
- Softened cream cheese

½ cup each:
- Splenda/your choice
- Walnuts/pecans

¼ cup brown sugar

4 tablespoons vanilla extract

Instructions
1. Wash and drain the grapes.
2. Combine the sour cream, cream cheese, vanilla, and sugar—blending well for about three to four minutes on high with a mixer.
3. Toss in the grapes and shake until covered.
4. Pour into a 9x13 cake pan. Sprinkle lightly with the brown sugar. Add the nuts.
5. Chill about one hour before serving.

Yields: 16 servings
Cal: 133.7 | P: 2.7 g | C: 18.4 g | F: 5.9 g

Israeli Salad

Ingredients

1 medium peeled cucumber
3 medium tomatoes
1 yellow/green bell pepper
3 tbsp. olive oil (extra-virgin is best)
2 tbsp. lemon juice
1 tsp. of each of pepper and salt

Instructions
1. Chop all of the veggies into small bits.
2. Mix everything together and enjoy.

Yields: Eight servings
Cal: 65.2 | P: 0.8 g | C: 4.4 g | F: 5.6g

Sunshine Fruit Salad

Ingredients
2 cans (15 ounces each) mandarin oranges in light syrup

3 cans (20 ounces each) pineapple chunks in 100% juice
2 large bananas
3 medium kiwi fruits – bite-sized

Instructions
1. Remove the liquid from the oranges and pineapple. Save the pineapple juice.
2. Combine all of the fruit (omit the bananas).
3. Submerge the fruit with the juice and chill for a minimum of one hour.
4. Slice and stir in the bananas before serving.

Yields: 10 servings
Cal: 135.2 | P: 1.5 g | C: 34.6 g | F: 0.4 g

Pasta Dishes

Skillet Lasagna

Ingredients
1 ¼ - cups water
1 small onion
3 minced cloves of garlic
8 ounces tomato sauce
1 lb. lean ground beef
1 can (14 ounces) diced tomatoes
2 ½ cups broken whole wheat lasagna noodles
1 teaspoon each:
- Oregano leaves
- Salt
- Basil leaves
- Parsley flakes

¼ cup grated fat-free parmesan cheese
1 egg
1 cup fat-free cottage cheese

Garnish: Mozzarella cheese
Optional: Pepper and dried basil

Instructions
1. Chop the onion. Brown the garlic, onions, and beef in a large frying pan. Remove the grease from the pan. Add the sauce, water, tomatoes, salt, oregano, basil, and parsley. Stir, add the noodles. Wait for it to boil.
2. Lower the heat and continue cooking, covered, for twenty minutes.
3. Blend in the parmesan and cottage cheese along with the egg.
4. Sprinkle with the pepper and basil.
5. Arrange a rounded tablespoon of the cheese mix onto the pasta.
6. Place a lid on the pot and cook five minutes. Sprinkle with some shredded mozzarella and enjoy.

Yields: Six servings
Cal: 342.3 | P: 28 g | C: 34.5 g | F: 10.7 g

Mediterranean Salmon with Pasta

Ingredients
4 (4 ounces) salmon fillets (16 ounces total)
2 medium sliced tomatoes
1 medium red bell pepper
4 cups whole wheat spaghetti - cooked
To Taste:
- Black pepper
- Lemon juice
2 tablespoons prepared pesto
Garnish: Drizzle of olive oil

Instructions

1. Slice the peppers into thin slices.
2. Program the oven setting to 400°F.
3. Arrange each of the fillets on the center of aluminum foil along with ½ tablespoon of the pesto sauce. Divide the veggies on/around the fish. Sprinkle with pepper and enclose the foil.
4. Bake 15 to 20 minutes.

Yields: Four servings
Cal: 407.5 | P: 38.7 g | C: 44.9 g | F: 9.2 g

Shrimp Pasta

Ingredients
8 ounces fettuccine
1 pound fresh medium shrimp
8 ounces of reduced-fat cream cheese
1 cup of each:
- Chicken broth
- Grated parmesan cheese

2 garlic cloves
5 ounces frozen spinach – thawed – moisture removed
To taste: Pepper and salt

Instructions
1. Prepare the fettuccine.
2. Heat a skillet using the med-high setting. Empty the chicken broth and cream cheese. Cook three to four minutes until the ingredients are well blended.
3. Add the garlic, pepper, and salt, along with the parmesan cheese.
4. Stir in the shrimp and stir until completely done. Toss in the spinach, stir, and enjoy.

Yields: Six servings
Cal: 363.5| P: 30.9g | C: 24.0 g | F: 15.2 g

Chapter 3: Lunch: Soups - Stews - and Sandwiches

Soups and Stews

Cabbage Vegetable Soup

Ingredients
1 medium diced onion
1 can each:
- 28 ounces - crushed tomatoes
- 14.5 ounces green beans
- 15 ounces can pinto beans
- 12 ounces sweet yellow corn

3 medium diced carrots
1 head shredded cabbage
3 diced stalks of celery

Instructions
1. Pour the tomatoes, cabbage, celery, onion, and carrots in a pot. Simmer about 20 minutes over medium heat.
2. Add the canned veggies and serve.

Yields: Six servings (1 ½ cups each)
Cal: 165.2 | P: 8.3 g | C: 36.6 g | F: 1.8 g

Chicken Tortilla Soup – Slow Cooker

Ingredients
1 lb. frozen chicken
1 can of:
- (15 oz.) whole tomatoes
- (4 oz.) chopped green chile peppers
- (15 oz.) black beans

- (10 oz.) enchilada sauce

1 medium onion

1 package (10 oz.) frozen corn

3 cans (14.5 oz.) chicken broth

2 minced garlic cloves

1 teaspoon cumin

¼ teaspoon black pepper

Instructions

1. Rinse the black beans.
2. Arrange the chicken, enchilada sauce, mashed tomatoes, chiles, chopped onions, and garlic into the crock pot.
3. Season the pot mixture with the pepper, salt, and cumin.
4. Pour in the chicken broth, black beans, and corn.
5. Cook low for six to eight hours or on high for three hours.
6. Top it off with some shredded cheese, avocados, sour cream or other ingredients of your choosing. Be sure to add the additional calories.

Yields: Eight servings

Cal: 169.1 | P: 17.4 g | C: 20.3 g | F: 2.5 g

Fifteen Minute Chili

Ingredients

½ cup chopped onions

1 pound ground turkey

1 can chopped stewed tomatoes (28 ounces)

1 can of each (16 ounces):

- Pinto beans
- Kidney beans

1 tablespoon each:

- Cumin powder
- Chili powder

½ cup salsa

Instructions

1. Rinse and drain the kidney and pinto beans.
2. Brown the onions and turkey in a large pot.
3. Empty the beans, tomatoes, cumin, chili powder, salsa, and garlic into the mixture. Cook until boiling and serve.
4. Garnish with some cheese (count the carbs).

Yields: Four servings
Cal: 370.8 | P: 31.3 g | C: 32.3 g | F: 13.3 g

5 Ingredient Soup

Ingredients
1 can each (14.4 ounces):
- Corn
- Fat-free chicken broth
- Diced tomatoes (no-salt added)
- Refried beans (fat-free)
- Black beans

Instructions

1. Rinse and drain the black beans and corn. In a medium pan, blend all of the ingredients using a whisk to blend in the refried beans.
2. Simmer and serve.
3. Garnish with some avocado, green onions, or sour cream.

Yields: Ten servings
Cal: 128.0 | P: 7.3 g | C: 24.9 g | F: 0.6 g

French Onion Soup

Ingredients
1 medium yellow onion
¼ cup water
4 cups beef broth

½ cup part-skim mozzarella cheese – shredded
2 slices whole-wheat bread

Instructions
1. Prepare a pot of boiling water.
2. Toss in the onion and continue cooking until the onions are translucent.
3. Pour in the beef broth and cook another 15 to 20 minutes
4. Add it to two cups. Garnish each one with one-ounce of shredded mozzarella and 1 tablespoon of croutons.
5. Place it under the broiler and melt the cheese, if you like it that way.

Yields: Two servings
Cal: 165.9 | P: 14.6 g | C: 14.7 g | F: 6.1 g

Potato Soup – Slow Cooker

Ingredients
3 large sliced carrots
6 large cubed potatoes
3 chopped celery stalks
2 chopped onions
4 chicken bouillon cubes
1 can - non-fat evaporated milk
6 cups of water
Optional: Shredded cheddar cheese (not in counts)

Instructions
1. Combine the veggies, water, and bouillon in a large slow cooker.
2. Use the high setting for three to four hours or the low for eight to ten hours.
3. Once the time has elapsed, add the milk and heat.
4. Serve and enjoy.

Yields: Twelve servings
Cal: 170.7 | P: 5.9 g | C: 36.7 g | F: 0.4 g

Tomato Soup

Ingredients
2 tbsp. olive oil
4 small slices of bread
1 cup onion
3 minced cloves of garlic
¼ tsp. red pepper flakes
2 pounds tomatoes
½ tsp. dried thyme
1 tbsp. brown sugar
1 tbsp. balsamic vinegar
1 ½ cups chicken stock

Instructions
1. Remove the seeds and chop the tomatoes. Finely chop the onion. Remove the crust from the bread.
2. Add the oil to a stock pot along with the garlic and onions. Saute five minutes.
3. Blend in the tomatoes, thyme, sugar, pepper, and bread. Cook for three minutes.
4. Puree with a food processor/immersion blender.
5. Slowly combine the stock and cook slowly for ten minutes. Pour in the vinegar and cook approximately 2 minutes.

Yields: Eight servings
Cal: 98.9 | P: 2.5 g | F: 4.1 g | C: 14.3 g

Sandwiches

BBQ Steak/Chicken Wrap

Ingredients
8 ounces sliced - cooked steak/chicken breast
2 cups baby spinach
4 whole wheat fat-free tortillas (8-inch)
1 cup of each:
- Frozen – thawed corn
- Can black beans

½ cup shredded cheese (low-fat cheddar)
¼ cup barbecue sauce

Instructions
1. Rinse and drain the beans.
2. Program the oven temperature to 400°F.
3. Use a small amount of cooking spray in a casserole dish.
4. Roll up each of the wraps and heat thoroughly for ten minutes.

Yields: Four servings
Cal: 405.5 | P: 31.5 g | C: 45.1 g | F: 11.4 g

Buffalo Chicken Sandwich

Ingredients
2 skinless chicken breasts (4 ounces each)
¼ cup each:
- Hot sauce
- Breadcrumbs

Pepper and salt to taste
1 tablespoon each:
- Vinegar
- Butter

Tomato and lettuce
2 whole grain hamburger buns

Instructions
1. Program the oven temperature setting to 450°F.
2. Combine the pepper, salt, and breadcrumbs.
3. Pound the meat with a mallet between some plastic to flatten it for even cooking.
4. Coat the chicken with the crumbs and arrange it on a lightly sprayed baking dish. Bake for 25 to 30 minutes.
5. In a plastic bag, add the butter, vinegar, and hot sauce along with the chicken. Shake to coat it evenly and add to the toasted buns.
6. Add the tomatoes and lettuce.
7. Add the extra calories if you add some dressing or mayo.

Yields: Two servings
Cal: 268.7 | P: 18.1 g | C: 34.3 g | F: 8.7 g

Cheesy Salsa Dog

Ingredients for the Black Bean Salsa:
1 cup diced tomatoes
½ cup each:
Frozen/canned corn
Black beans – drained and rinsed
1 teaspoon cumin seeds
1 jalapeno - chopped
1 lime – zested and juiced
½ teaspoon chili powder
2 tablespoons chopped cilantro

Other Ingredients
¼ cup sharp cheddar cheese (shredded reduced-fat)
4 each:

- Whole wheat hot dog buns
- Turkey/soy hot dogs

Instructions
1. Remove the seeds along with the ribs from the jalapeno if you want to lower the heat factor.
2. Set the oven temperature to 400°F.
3. Mix all of the ingredients for the salsa.
4. Arrange the hot dogs on a pan and roast 15 minutes.
5. Over med-high heat, spray the buns with a small amount of cooking spray and arrange in a skillet. Toast until browned and add ¼ of the mixture to each of the buns.

Yields: Four servings
Cal: 194.7 | P: 14 g | C: 34.7 g | F: 2.6 g

Crab Melt

Ingredients
2 hard-boiled chopped egg whites
12 ounces imitation crabmeat (coarsely chopped)
2 tablespoons chopped onion
4 tablespoons light mayonnaise
Dash of black pepper
¼ cup shredded Swiss cheese
4 slices of each:
- ¼-inch tomatoes
- Whole-wheat bread

Instructions
- Mix the crab, egg whites, and onion, pepper, and mayonnaise.
- Arrange the sliced of bread on the broiler pan topping with the tomatoes, crab, and mayo mixture.
- Sprinkle each one with the Swiss cheese and broil.

- *Note*: You can use real crab but would need to adjust the counts.

Yields: Four servings
Cal: 296.3 | P: 20.3 g | C: 32.4 g | F: 9.6 g

Hawaiian Turkey Burger

Ingredients
40 ounces ground turkey
1 can (20 ounces) pineapple in unsweetened juice
2 tablespoons each:
- Minced garlic
- Ketchup
1 tablespoon each:
- Black pepper
- White vinegar
¼ teaspoon each:
- Red pepper flakes
- Salt
6 slices turkey bacon

Instructions
1. Dice the bacon into small bits and cook in a pan. Set aside in a dish.
2. Drain the juice from the pineapples and set aside.
3. Combine the turkey, ¾ cup of the crushed pineapple, pepper, and salt in a large mixing dish.
4. In another dish, combine the ketchup, pepper flakes, pineapple juice, vinegar, and soy sauce.
5. Form the patties into 24 portions and add in a single layer to a casserole dish. Pour the pineapple juice mixture over the patties and refrigerate, covered for about an hour, turning after 30 minutes.

6. Cook the patties on a George Forman grill for two minutes or one minute on each side on a regular grill.

Yields: 24 servings
Cal: 92 | P: 9.4 g | C: 3.1 g | F: 4.1 g

Ranch Cheddar Turkey Burgers

Ingredients
1 (one ounce) pouch dry ranch dressing mix
¼ cup chopped scallion
1 cup shredded cheese (low-fat)
1 lb. lean ground turkey

Instructions
1. Mix all of the fixings and form six patties.
2. Cook on the grill/skillet about six to seven minutes for each side.
3. Enjoy with tomato and lettuce on a bun (not included on counts).

Yields: Six servings
Cal: 155.1 | P: 19.3 g | C: 3.6 g | F: 6.7 g

Vegetarian Philly Cheese steak Sandwich

Ingredients
4 teaspoons minced garlic
1 green pepper
1 medium yellow onion
2 tablespoons light whipped salad dressing
1 slice each low-fat:
   ▪ American cheese
   ▪ Cheddar cheese
2 whole wheat burger buns

¼ cup sliced button mushrooms

Instructions
1. Slice the onion and green pepper into chunks.
2. Lightly spray a skillet and heat on the medium-low setting. Add the onions, peppers, and minced garlic. Add a pinch of pepper, stir the veggies, and cover. Sauté for several minutes.
3. Blend in the mushrooms and sauté for a couple for two or three minutes.
4. Cut the cheeses into quarters and spread out over the veggies over low heat.
5. Add the dressing to the buns and the ingredients, close and enjoy.

Yields: One serving
Cal: 274.7 | P: 27.5 g | C: 77.6 g | F: 13.6 g

Chapter 4: Dinner Dishes

Chicken Broccoli and Tomato Stir Fry

Ingredients
1 lb. breast of chicken
1 tbsp. soy sauce
¼ teaspoon salt
2 tsp. canola oil
1 tsp. fresh ginger
2 tsp. finely chopped garlic
3 cups broccoli florets
4 firm plum tomatoes (quartered lengthwise)
1 cup (divided) reduced-sodium chicken broth
1 tbsp. cornstarch

Instructions
1. Remove any bones and cut the chicken into one-inch chunks. Finely chop the ginger.
2. Use a wok or 12-inch skillet over the med-high setting to warm the oil. Toss in the chopped breast of chicken and cook three minutes.
3. Pour in the soy sauce, ginger, and garlic. Stir and mix in the broccoli and ½ cup of the chicken broth. Cover and cook two to three more minutes.
4. Mix the remainder of the broth and cornstarch until dissolved. Add it and the tomatoes to the skillet.
5. Lower the heat to med-low and simmer two minutes.

Yields: Four servings
Cal: 177.8 | P: 18.7 g | C: 22.1 g | F: 1.8 g

Chicken and Broccoli Casserole

Ingredients
1 lb. chicken breasts
10 ounces frozen broccoli spears
3 tbsp. mayonnaise
1 can cream of mushroom soup
1 cup cheddar cheese

Instructions
1. Use fat-free and low-sodium products.
2. Boil and drain the chicken breasts. When cooled, cut into one-inch bits, and remove any skin or bones.
3. Add the soup and mayonnaise in a casserole dish. Blend in the chicken and broccoli, mixing well.
4. Sprinkle the casserole with the shredded cheese.
5. Bake for approximately 20 minutes or until nicely browned.

Yields: Four servings
Cal: 284.2 | P: 36.8 g | C: 15.8 g | F: 7.3 g

Beef

Bavarian Beef

Ingredients
1 tbsp. olive oil
1 ¼ pounds stewing beef
1 large onion
¾ tsp. caraway seeds
½ tsp. salt
1 ½ - cups water
Pinch of black pepper
1 bay leaf

1 tbsp. sugar
¼ cup vinegar
½ small head of cabbage
¼ cup crushed gingersnaps

Instructions
1. Slice the beef into one-inch chunks. Thinly slice the onion. Cut the cabbage into four wedges.
2. Brown the beef in a skillet using the oil. Remove and drain the meat. Sauté the onion until lightly browned. Place the meat back into the skillet.
3. Pour in the water, bay leaf, pepper, salt, and caraway seeds.
4. When it starts to boil, lower the temperature, and continue cooking for 1 ¼ hours.
5. Pour in the sugar and vinegar. Stir and add the cabbage on top of the meat. Simmer the ingredients covered for another 45 minutes.
6. Transfer the cabbage and meat to a platter.
7. Strain the drippings and add enough water to make one cup of juices. Pour in the gingersnaps to the skillet and cook until thickened.
8. Serve the sauce over the meat and veggies.

Yields: Five servings (5 ounces each portion)
Cal: 256.1 | P: 29.1 g | C: 12.1 g | F: 10.1 g

BBQ Steak/Chicken Wrap

Ingredients
8 ounces sliced - cooked steak/chicken breast
2 cups baby spinach
4 whole wheat fat-free tortillas (8-inch)
1 cup of each:
   ▪ Frozen – thawed corn

- Can black beans

½ cup shredded cheese (low-fat cheddar)

¼ cup barbecue sauce

Instructions
1. Rinse and drain the beans.
2. Program the oven temperature setting to 400°F.
3. Spray a baking dish with a small amount of oil.
4. Roll up each of the wraps and heat thoroughly for ten minutes.

Yields: Four servings

Cal: 405.5 | P: 31.5 g | C: 45.1 g | F: 11.4 g

DC Sloppy Joes

Ingredients

16 ounces ground beef

1 cup diet cola

2 tablespoons each:
- Dry mustard
- White vinegar

1 tablespoon Worcestershire sauce

Garlic powder

Instructions
1. Brown the beef in a skillet, drain, and place it back into the pan.
2. Stir in the remainder of the fixings and stir.
3. Cook uncovered on the low setting for 30 minutes.

Yields: Four servings

Cal: 162.5| P: 24.0g | C: 2.5 g | F: 4.5 g

Ginger Beef

Ingredients
1 pound flank steak
2 tablespoons each:
- Seasoned rice vinegar
- Lite soy sauce

2 teaspoons each:
- Corn starch
- Ground ginger

½ cup water
1 teaspoon garlic powder
10 slices fresh ginger root (1-inch diameter)
8 large scallions

Instructions
1. Slice the ginger into wafer thin slices, and dice. Wash and slice the scallions.
2. Mix the garlic powder, ground ginger, water, soy sauce, and vinegar.
3. Slice the meat into one-inch strips against the grain of the meat. Chill in the fridge for about 20 minutes.
4. Spray a skillet/wok with non-stick cooking oil. Using the high setting, add the veggies and meat. It should take about ten minutes to brown.
5. At the end of the cooking cycle; mix the corn starch in some water and stir quickly into the juices to thicken.

Yields: Four servings
Cal: 207.6| P: 22.9 g | C: 10.3 g | F: 8.0 g

Ground Beef Casserole - Keema

Ingredients
1 ½ pounds lean ground sirloin

2 cups crushed tomatoes
1 cup of each:
- Chopped onions
- Diced potatoes
- Frozen peas

1 tablespoon curry powder
½ teaspoon each:
- Ginger
- Turmeric
- Cinnamon

Pepper and salt if desired

Instructions
1. Brown the onions and sirloin in a pan. Add the potatoes peas, tomatoes, and spices.
2. Simmer for 25 minutes adding a pinch of pepper and salt.
3. It should look like chili.

Yields: Six servings
Cal: 197.3 | P: 22.4 g | C: 11.6 g | F: 7.0 g

Ground Beef and Potato Casserole

Ingredients
1 can (10 ¾ oz.) Healthy Quest by Campbell's Cream of Mushroom Soup
¼ cup water
1 cup chopped onions
3-4 medium potatoes
1 lb. lean ground beef
¼ teaspoon each:
- Black pepper
- Salt (optional)

Instructions
1. Program the oven to 350°F.
2. Prepare the potatoes thinly sliced with skins left on.
3. Brown the onions and beef; drain.
4. In a 9x11-inch (2 quart) casserole dish, lightly spray, and alternate layers of potatoes with layers of beef.
5. Pour ½ of the soup mixture over this and add an additional layer with the rest of the ingredients.
6. Bake one hour.

Yields: Six to eight servings
Cal: 166.3 | P: 14.0 g | C: 18.5 g | F: 4.1 g

Mushroom and Beef - Slow Cooker

Ingredients
1 pound lean stewing beef
1 pouch dry onion soup mix
½ cup water
1 can - cream of mushroom soup (low-fat)
8 ounces fresh sliced/whole mushrooms

Instructions
1. Use a pan on the medium heat setting to cook the meat, and add it to the slow cooker (4-quart is best).
2. Add the meat in the bottom and the mushrooms. Mix the soup mix water, and can of soup together and pour into the pot.
3. Serve over some noodles or brown rice. (Count the calories.)

Yields: Four servings
Cal: 410.5| P: 34.8 g | C: 12.4 g | F: 23.9 g

Slimmer Beef Stroganoff - Stir Fry

Ingredients
1 ½ - cups whole wheat bow tie pasta
1 pound beef tenderloin tips
1/3 cup chopped onion
½ pound sliced mushrooms
2 teaspoons olive oil
1 can (10.5 ounces) beef broth
2 tablespoons whole wheat flour

Instructions
1. Prepare the pasta.
2. Cut the beef into one inch cubes and trim away all fat.
3. Lightly grease a skillet with a small amount of cooking spray. Combine the beef, and stir fry for three to five minutes on the medium heat setting. Transfer to a dish.
4. In the same pan add the oil, onions, and mushrooms. Cook for two to three minutes.
5. Blend in the flour and broth stirring until blended.
6. Once it begins to boil cook for about two minutes. Add pepper and salt.

Yields: One serving
Cal: 514.5| P: 30.9 g | C: 42.4 g | F: 24.1 g

Chicken and Turkey

Baked Chicken and Vegetables

Ingredients
6 sliced carrots
4 sliced potatoes
1 large quartered onion
1 skinless raw chicken

1 teaspoon thyme
½ cup water
¼ teaspoon pepper

Instructions
1. Program the temperature of the oven in advance to 400°F.
2. Arrange the carrots, potatoes, and onions in a large roasting pan. Add the chicken last.
3. Combine the thyme, pepper, and water. Empty the mixture over the ingredients in the pan.
4. Place in the oven to bake for one hour until brown and tender. Baste the chicken with the juices several times.

Yields: Six servings
Cal: 240 | P: 26 g | C: 25 g | F: 3.5g

Brown Sugar Garlic Chicken

Ingredients
12 ounces chicken breasts (no skin or bones)
1 garlic clove
2 tbsp. butter
Dash of black pepper

Instructions
1. Melt the butter and add the garlic in a frying pan.
2. Add the chicken seasoning with the pepper and cook until done. It usually takes approximately 15 minutes.
3. Sprinkle the chicken with the brown sugar and cook for five minutes and serve.

Yields: Four servings
Cal: 166.4 | P: 19.4 g | C: 4.3 g | F: 8.0 g

Chicken Creole

Ingredients
4 chicken breasts – 1-inch strips – skinless and boneless
1 cup low-sodium chili sauce
1 can cut up tomatoes (14 ounces)
¼ cup onion
½ cup celery
1 ½ cups green peppers (1 large)
2 minced garlic cloves
1 tablespoon fresh each:
- Parsley
- Basil

¼ teaspoon each:
- Crushed red pepper
- Salt

Instructions
1. Chop the celery, onion, and green peppers.
2. Lightly grease a frying pan with some cooking spray.
3. Warm the pan on the high setting. Cook the chicken for three to five minutes.
4. Lower the temperature and combine the remainder of the ingredients.
5. Once it starts to boil, put a top on the pan, and cook slowly for about ten minutes.
6. You can enjoy this tasty meal over a bed of rice (calories not included in counts).

Yields: One serving
Cal: 269.3| P: 32.8 g | C: 20.7 g | F: 6.3 g

Chicken Enchiladas and Sour Cream

Ingredients
½ can (14.5 ounces) each:
- Fat-free cream of chicken soup
- Mexican Rotel

1 cup sour cream - fat-free
12 ounces cooked shredded chicken breast
½ chopped white/yellow onion
1 tablespoon fresh chopped cilantro
16 corn tortillas
1 cup shredded Colby/pepper jack cheese blend (reduced-fat)

Instructions
1. Mix the soup, sour cream, and cilantro in a saucepan. Heat and set to the side.
2. Lightly grease a pan with a small amount of cooking spray. Blend the Rotel, chicken, and onions into the pan.
3. Warm the tortillas in the microwave until they are flexible.
4. Divide all of the ingredients between the tortillas and add them to a casserole dish.
5. Pour the cream sauce over the tortillas along with the rest of the cheese.

Yields: Eight servings (2 enchiladas each)
Cal: 252.0 | P: 18.3 g | C: 35.0 g | F: 4.5 g

Chicken Tetrazzini

Ingredients
1 tbsp. reduced calorie margarine
8 ounces sliced button mushrooms
½ cup chopped scallions – approximately 5
¼ tsp. garlic powder

3 tbsp. all-purpose flour
1 pinch of black pepper
1 cup chicken broth (fat-free)
½ pounds chicken breasts
½ cup skim milk
¼ cup pimentos (2 ounce jar)
2 tbsp. sherry cooking wine
8 ounces uncooked spaghetti
3 ½ tbsp. grated parmesan cheese

Instructions
1. Break the spaghetti into thirds, cook, and drain. Cook and cube the breasts.
2. Add the margarine, scallions, and mushrooms into a large pan. Sauté for approximately five minutes.
3. Blend the flour, garlic powder, pepper, milk and broth together in a small mixing container. Add in the mixture and continue cooking until thickened, usually about ten minutes.
4. Blend in the chicken, sherry, and pimentos. Cook about two minutes.
5. Stir in the cheese and cooked spaghetti.

Yields: Six servings (one cup each)
Cal: 167 | P: 10 g | C: 25g | F: 3 g

Cola Chicken

Ingredients
3 chicken breasts
1 cup ketchup
1 can (12 ounces) diet cola
Garnish: Chopped green onion

Instructions

1. Arrange the chicken in a skillet and pour in the cola and ketchup.
2. Place a lid on the skillet and let the ingredients start to boil. Lower the heat setting, and continue cooking slowly for about 45 minutes.
3. Uncover and raise the temperature until the sauce thickens and begins to stick to the chicken.

Yields: Three servings
Cal: 193.8| P: 16.2g | C: 21.4 g | F: 1.9 g

Creamy Italian Chicken – Slow Cooker

Ingredients
2 pounds chicken breasts (no skin or bones)
½ cup water
1 - 8 ounce package of reduced-fat cream cheese
1 pouch Italian dressing mix
1 can cream of chicken soup
3 cups long grain rice – cooked – brown or white

Instructions

1. Arrange the chicken in the crock pot.
2. Combine the water and dressing mixture. Pour it over the chicken.
3. Put the lid on the cooker and let it cook on low for eight hours or high for four hours. Transfer the chicken to a plate.
4. In a separate dish, add the soup and cream cheese. Pour the mixture into the pot. Add all ingredients back into the cooker as you gently shred the chicken.
5. Continue cooking on low until all ingredients are heated.
6. Serve with the rice.

For Best Results: Use the lower setting so all ingredients fully integrated.

Yields: Six servings (2/3 cup chicken with ½ cup of rice)
Cal: 385.4 | P: 41.0 g | C: 24.1 g | F: 12.5 g

Fish

BBQ Roasted Salmon

Ingredients
4 (6 ounces) salmon fillets
2 tablespoons fresh lemon juice
¼ cup pineapple juice

Instructions
1. Program the oven temperature to 400°F.
2. Add the first three ingredients into a Ziploc plastic bag. Marinate for a minimum of one hour—turning occasionally.
3. Remove the salmon and throw the marinade in the trash.
4. Combine the rest of the ingredients and rub it over the fish.
5. Arrange them in a lightly coated baking dish for 12 to 15 minutes.
6. Garnish with some lemon.

Yields: Four servings
Cal: 225 | P: 34 g | C: 7 g | F: 6 g

Breaded Cod Fillet

Ingredients
4 (6 ounces) skinless cod
Non-stick cooking spray

¼ teaspoon black pepper
¾ teaspoon fine sea salt
3 tablespoons –divided-unsalted melted margarine
¼ cup dried whole wheat bread crumbs
Juice of 1 lemon – divided
2 tablespoons chopped chives
3 tablespoons finely chopped parsley
Also Needed: 9 x 13 baking dish

Instructions
1. Program the oven to 425°F.
2. Lightly coat the baking dish with cooking spray.
3. Flavor the cod with the pepper and salt and place in the dish.
4. Drizzle half of the lemon juice and margarine over the fish.
5. Mix the chives, parsley, and breadcrumbs in a bowl. Sprinkle it over the cod along with the remainder of lemon and margarine.
6. Bake for approximately 12 minutes.

Yields: Four servings (six ounces each)
Cal: 150 | P: 11 g | C: 6 g | F: 9 g

Broiled Tilapia Parmesan

Ingredients
1 tbsp. fresh lemon juice
2 tbsp. softened butter
1 tbsp. (+) 1 ½ tsp. reduced fat mayonnaise
1 pound tilapia fillets
1/8 tsp. each of:
- Ground black pepper
- Dried basil
- Onion powder

- Celery seed

Instructions
1. Preheat the broiler on the oven. Line with foil or grease a broiling pan.
2. Combine the butter, mayonnaise, parmesan cheese, and lemon juice in a small container. Add the onion powder, pepper, basil, and celery salt. Stir and set to the side.
3. Place the fillets into the baking pan and broil two to three minutes. Flip them once and broil two additional minutes.
4. Take the fish out of the oven and coat them with the cheese mixture. Broil two more minutes.

Yields: Four servings
Cal: 177.1 | P: 19.6 g | C: 1.2 g | F: 10.5g

Mock Crab Cakes

Ingredients
2 egg whites
2 pounds imitation crabmeat
1 sleeve (34) Keebler Toasteds/or other crackers – crushed
4 tablespoons light mayonnaise

Instructions
1. Warm up the oven in advance to 375°F.
2. Whisk the eggs until fluffy and blend in the mayonnaise
3. Add the crushed crackers with the eggs and combine with the crabmeat.
4. Make the patties using about ½- cup for each patty.
5. Bake 15 minutes per side.

Yields: 10 servings
Cal: 161.4 | P: 7.4 g | C: 21.6 g | F: 4.4 g

Oven-Fried Tilapia

Ingredients
3 egg whites
One pound (4) tilapia fillets
1 tablespoon each:
- Onion powder
- Garlic powder
- Grated parmesan cheese
- Cajun seasoning

1 ½ cups finely ground Fiber One cereal/oven-fry bread
Non-stick cooking spray

Instructions
1. Program the oven temperature to 400°F.
2. Whisk the egg whites until frothy.
3. In a separate container, combine all of the seasonings, cheese, and cereal.
4. Lightly spray a cookie sheet and add the fish. Spritz a small amount of oil directly on the fish.
5. Bake 8 to 10 minutes.

Yields: Four servings (4 ounces each)
Cal: 184.7 | P: 27.9 g | C: 22.1 g | F: 3.1 g

Salmon - Quick and Easy

Ingredients
12 ounces fresh salmon
¼ cup each soy sauce
Maple syrup/honey (not pancake syrup)
2-3 minced garlic cloves

Instructions

1. Combine all of the fixings into a Ziploc bag and shake. Place the salmon into the marinade, and refrigerate for at least an hour.
2. Add all of the components into a casserole dish, and cover with aluminum foil.
3. Lastly, place the salmon into the oven and bake for 15 minutes at 350°F.

Yields: Four servings (3 ounces each)
Cal: 183.1 | P: 18.0 g | C: 14.9 g | F: 5.5 g

Salmon Patties

Ingredients
¼ cup green bell pepper
½ medium onion
1 celery stalk
1 can pink salmon
½ cup breadcrumbs
1 egg
½ teaspoon each:
- Chili powder
- *Optional*: Old Bay Seasoning

Instructions
1. Chop the pepper, onion, and celery into fine bits.
2. Clean the salmon by discarding the bones and skin.
3. Mix the egg, veggies, breadcrumbs, salmon, and seasonings together.
4. Scoop them out and add to a well-greased griddle.
5. Smash the patty and cook five minutes per side.
6. Top with a bit of ketchup or horseradish.

Yields: Four servings
Cal: 216.8 | P: 25.8 g | C: 10.5 g | F: 7.8 g

Pork

Asian Pork Tenderloin

Ingredients
1/3 cup each of:
- Brown sugar
- Light soy sauce

2 tablespoons each:
- Rice vinegar
- Worcestershire sauce
- Lemon juice

1 tablespoon each of:
- Ginger
- Dry mustard

1 ½ teaspoons pepper
4 minced garlic cloves
2 lbs. pork tenderloin

Instructions
1. Program the oven to 375°F.
2. Add all of the ingredients into a freezer bag along with the tenderloin.
3. Place in the fridge overnight.
4. Bake for 30 to 40 minutes.
5. *Note*: You can also use the slow cooker for four to six hours.

Yields: Eight servings (4 ounces each)
Cal: 256 | P: 34 g | C: 9 g | F: 9 g

BBQ Pulled Pork Roast – Slow Cooker

Ingredients
1 cup each:
- Chopped onions

- Chopped celery
- Water
- Barbecue sauce
- Ketchup

2 tablespoons each:
- Worcestershire sauce
- Brown sugar
- Vinegar

1 teaspoon each:
- Chili powder
- Salt

½ teaspoon each:
- Pepper
- Garlic powder

3 pounds boneless pork roast

Instructions
1. Mix all of the ingredients in the slow cooker.
2. Arrange the roast in the pot last.
3. Cover and cook for six to seven hours on high.
4. Transfer the meat to a platter, shred, and return to the pot.
5. Simmer until hot and enjoy.

Yields: 12 servings
Cal: 296.9 | P: 32.4 g | C: 12.3 g | F: 11.9 g

Grilled Honey Garlic Pork Chops

Ingredients
3 tablespoons soy sauce
¼ (+) 1/8 cup honey
6 boneless fat-free pork loin chops
6 minced garlic cloves

Instructions
1. Blend the soy sauce, garlic, and honey. Evenly cover the chops.
2. Save the honey mix for basting.
3. Grill over med-high heat with a closed lid.

Yields: Six servings
Cal: 204.3 | P: 19.9 g | C: 18.4 g | F: 5.7 g

Mustard Brown Sugar Pork Chops

Ingredients
1/3 cup yellow mustard
½ cup brown sugar
6 boneless pork loin chops

Instructions
1. Blend the sugar and mustard together and pour over the chops.
2. Bake 25 minutes at 350°F.

Yields: Six servings
Cal: 228.1| P: 20.7 g | C: 24.6 g | F: 7.8 g

Chapter 5: Veggie Dishes

Black Bean and Rice Casserole

Ingredients
1/3 cup diced onion
1 cup vegetable broth
1/3 cup brown rice
1 tbsp. olive oil
1 lb. chopped chicken breast (no skin or bones)
1 medium thinly sliced zucchini
½ cup sliced mushrooms
¼ tsp. cayenne pepper
½ tsp. cumin
1 can (4 ounces) diced green chilies
1 can (15 ounces) drained black beans
1/3 cup shredded carrots
2 cups −divided - shredded Swiss cheese

Instructions
1. Prepare a pot with the vegetable broth and rice. Let the pan start a gentle boiling and lower the heat setting. Cook covered on low for 45 minutes.
2. Program the oven temperature to 350°F.
3. Spray a baking dish with some cooking spray.
4. Warm the oil in a pan using the medium heat setting. Toss in the onion and cook until tender. Add the chicken, zucchini, mushrooms, and seasonings. Continue cooking until the chicken is heated and the zucchini is lightly browned.
5. In a mixing dish, blend in the onion, cooked rice, chicken, zucchini, beans, chilies, mushrooms, one cup of Swiss cheese, and the carrots.
6. Empty the ingredients into the casserole dish along with the remainder of the Swiss cheese as a topping. Cover and

bake 30 minutes. Uncover, and continue cooking ten more minutes.

Yields: Eight servings
Cal: 267| P: 31 g | C: 22 g | F: 6 g

Broccoli Casserole

Ingredients
4 cups cut up broccoli
1 sleeve Ritz crackers
2 cups cheddar cheese

Instructions
1. Add the casserole ingredients into a Pyrex dish with the crumbled crackers on top.
2. Bake long enough to melt the cheese at 375°F.

Yields: 12 servings
Cal: 90.5 | P: 10.3 g | C: 9.8 g | F: 2.3 g

Eggplant Pesto Mini Pizza

Ingredients
1 each chopped:
- Bell pepper
- Tomato
- Eggplant

1 medium sliced red onion
1/8 teaspoon salt
3 cloves of garlic
Pinch of oregano
¼ cup each:
- Extra-virgin olive oil
- Pesto sauce

- Hummus

Vegan Parmesan cheese

Sandwich thins – Arnold Orowheat used

Optional: Pepper flakes

Instructions
1. Set the oven to 400°F.
2. Chop the vegetables and combine with the oil, pepper, salt, oregano, and pepper flakes if desired. Arrange on a cookie tin and toast for approximately 30 to 45 minutes.
3. Toast the buns and spread the hummus on them, add the veggies, and a bit of pesto sauce. Sprinkle with the vegan cheese and enjoy.

Yields: Four servings

Cal: 405| P: 11.4 g | C: 40.6 g | F: 24.5 g

Quinoa and Black Bean Casserole

Ingredients

2 cans (15 ounces) black beans

1 cup cooked quinoa

2 large shredded sweet potatoes

1 cup (divided) shredded low-fat cheddar cheese

Pinches of pepper and salt

1 tablespoon ground cumin

1 cup salsa

2 eggs

Garnish: 2 tablespoons cilantro – chopped

Instructions
1. Program the oven setting temperature to 350°F.
2. Lightly spray a square casserole dish (9x9).
3. Combine the beans, potatoes, quinoa, ½ - cup of the cheese, pepper, salt, and cumin.

4. Mix the salsa and eggs and combine everything into the casserole dish.
5. Add the remainder of the cheese for the top layer and bake for 30 minutes – uncovered.

Yields: Eight servings (one-cup each)
Cal: 204.5 | P: 13.8 g | C: 31.7 g | F: 3.2 g

Vegetable Curry – Slow Cooker

Ingredients
2 cups sliced carrots
1 tbsp. canola oil
1 onion
3 cloves of garlic
2 tbsp. curry powder
1 tsp. ground cumin
½ tsp. each:
- Turmeric
- Garam masala

8 ounces fresh/frozen green beans
4-5 potatoes – quartered
1 cup/2 large diced tomatoes
3 cups chickpeas (canned- drained-rinsed)
2 cups vegetable stock
½ cup each:
- Frozen peas
- Light coconut milk

Instructions
1. Slice the carrots about 1/3 inches thick. Thinly slice the onion and garlic.
2. Warm the oil and toss in the onions and carrots, sautéing for about three to four minutes. Add the cumin, curry

powder, garlic, turmeric, and garam masala to the pan and cook two more minutes.

3. Transfer the veggies to the slow cooker. Add the green beans, potatoes, chick peas, vegetable stock, and chick peas to the cooker.

4. Set the timer for 5 ½ hours on the low setting. After that time elapses, add the peas and milk cooking 15 more minutes.

Yields: Eight servings (one cup each)
Cal: 183.6 | P: 7 g | C: 30.5 g | F: 3.8 g

Vegetarian Chili

Ingredients
1 can (15 ounces) each:
- Black beans
- Pinto beans
- Dark red kidney beans
- Light red kidney beans

1 can (28 ounces) diced tomatoes
2 cans (28 ounces) crushed tomatoes
3 cups celery
1 small diced each of red and yellow bell peppers
1 medium red onion
4 tbsp. chili powder
2 tbsp. ground cumin
3 tbsp. garlic powder

Instructions
1. Drain and rinse all of the beans. Dice the veggies.
2. Lightly spray a large pan over medium heat and cook the veggies about six to seven minutes or until they are softened.

3. Combine the spices, beans, and tomatoes in a slow cooker or a Dutch oven.

Yields: Eight servings
Cal: 279.8 | P: 14.7 g | C: 58.4 g | F: 2.2 g

Vegetarian Lentil Loaf

Ingredients
1 ½ cups rinsed – dried lentils
2 yellow onions
3 cups cooked brown rice
2 tablespoons canola/olive oil
½ cup of ketchup
1 can of (6 oz.) tomato paste
1 teaspoon each of:
- Garlic powder
- Sage
- Marjoram

½ cup - quartered cherry tomatoes
¾ cup tomato/pasta sauce
To Taste:
- Salt
- More ketchup

Instructions
1. Program the oven temperature to 350°F.
2. Rinse and cook the lentils in 3 to 4 cups of water for approximately 30 minutes.
3. Drain and slightly mash the lentils.
4. Peel and chop the onions. Cook in the oil until golden.
5. Combine the onions, lentils, tomato paste, rice, tomatoes, sauce and spices into a large pot. Mix well.
6. Press the mixture into a well-greased baking dish with ½ cup of ketchup over the top.

7. Bake for one hour.

Yields: Ten servings
Cal: 254.2| P: 10.9 g | C: 44.9 g | F: 4.4 g

Veggie Frittata

Ingredients
6 ounces button mushrooms
1 pound asparagus
1 shallot
1 clove of garlic
1 small zucchini
1 tablespoon olive oil
6 large eggs
1/3 cup 1% milk
1 teaspoon salt
¼ teaspoon of black pepper
1 tablespoon chopped chives
Dash of nutmeg
2 medium/1 large tomato
¼ cup freshly grated parmesan cheese

Instructions
1. Program the oven temperature ahead of time to 350°F.
2. *Prepare the asparagus*: Wash and trim cutting it into one-inch pieces. Blanche the cut asparagus for one to two minutes. Shock it by adding it to ice water. Drain and set to the side.
3. Wash and slice the mushrooms. Sauté them in the oil for ten minutes using medium heat. Mince the shallots and garlic and add – cooking two more minutes. Transfer the mushrooms to a plate.
4. Slice the zucchini lengthwise and slice again to create half-moon shapes.

5. Whisk the eggs, milk, chives, pepper, salt, and nutmeg in a large mixing dish. Add the mushrooms, zucchini, and asparagus.
6. Add the egg/veggie mixture to a lightly greased 2-quart baking dish.
7. Arrange the thinly sliced tomatoes on top and sprinkle with the parmesan cheese.
8. Bake 30-35 minutes. You can place the frittata under the broiler for two to three minutes to brown the top.
9. Cool and serve at room temperature or straight from the fridge.

Yields: Six servings
Cal: 146.2 | P: 10.6 g | C: 7.4 g | F: 8.8 g

Chapter 6: Snacks, Desserts, and Drinks

Snacks

Cheese Quesadilla

Ingredients
1/3 cup Mexican shredded blend cheese
Low-carb/Low-fat wrap (13 g. carbs in Toufayan used in recipe)
1 tablespoon sour cream (full-fat)
2 tablespoons salsa
1 tablespoon /½ pat salted butter

Instructions
1. Lightly butter the wrap and set it butter side down on the griddle/frying pan.
2. Add the cheese (1/4-inch from the edge)
3. Cover and wait for the cheese to melt, close and cook until crispy brown; flip and do the other side.
4. Cut into 3 wedges and add the toppings desired.

Yields: One serving
Cal: 298.2 | P: 23 g | C: 18.8 g | F: 14.2 g

Chili Popcorn

Ingredients
½ tablespoon melted margarine
1-quart popped popcorn
¼ teaspoon ground cumin
1 ¼ teaspoons chili powder
A dash of garlic powder

Instructions
1. Pop the corn and add the margarine.
2. Combine the seasonings and add over the popcorn.
3. Shake well and enjoy

Yields: Four servings /one-cup each
Cal: 45.7 | P: 1.1 g | C: 6.7 g | F: 1.9 g

Hummus

Ingredients
¼ each:
- Sesame paste – tahini
- Water

2 cups garbanzo beans/chickpeas
3 tablespoons each:
- Olive oil
- Fresh lemon juice

¾ teaspoons salt
1 tablespoon ground cumin

Instructions
1. Rinse and drain the chickpeas.
2. Combine all of the fixings into a food processor or blender until creamy smooth.
3. Store the hummus in a closed container for a maximum of seven to ten days.

Yields: Six servings
Cal: 215.9 | P: 5.8 g | C: 21.2 g | F: 12.8 g

Roasted Kale Chips

Ingredients
1 tablespoon olive oil
1 bunch of kale
 Salt to your liking

Instructions
1. Set the oven temperature to 350°F.
2. Place a piece of parchment paper on a baking sheet.
3. Remove the kale stem and make sure it's completely dry.
4. Sprinkle the kale with salt and the incorporate the oil.
5. Lay them singly on the baking sheet and roast about 15 minutes, or until crunchy and slightly browned.
6. Cool them and enjoy.

Yields: Four servings
Cal: 66.2 | P: 2.5 g | C: 7.3 g | F: 3.9 g

Desserts - Sweet Snacks

Banana Nut Granola

Ingredients
1 small ripe banana
1 cup raw almonds
½ cup honey/maple syrup
5 cups old-fashioned oats
3 cups barley flakes
½ cup each:
- Ground flaxseed
- Unsweetened coconut (optional)

1 tablespoon ground cinnamon

Instructions

1. Program the oven temperature to 350°F.
2. Process the almonds until they are finely ground (around two minutes) in a food processor.
3. Add the syrup and banana, processing another minute until pourable.
4. Add the barley and oats in a large container and pour in the banana mixture.
5. Spread out on the baking sheet and bake for thirty minutes. Stir every ten minutes.

Yields: 16 servings - ½ cup each
Cal: 248.9 | P: 7.6 g | C: 35.9 g | F: 9.4 g

Caramel Popcorn

Ingredients
1 cup packed dark brown sugar
½ cup light-colored corn syrup
¼ cup butter
½ teaspoon each:
- Baking soda
- Salt

1 ½ teaspoons vanilla extract
7 tablespoons kernels - 12 cups air-popped popcorn

Instructions
1. Set the oven temperature to 250°F.
2. Coat a jelly roll pan with a small amount of cooking spray.
3. In a heavy-bottomed saucepan, add the butter, corn syrup, and sugar, bringing it to a boil. Cook over medium heat for four to five minutes.
4. Take the pan from the heat source and blend in the salt, baking soda, and vanilla.
5. Use a large bowl for the popcorn and pour the melted mixture over the kernels, stirring to coat evenly.

6. Add this to the pan and bake 45 minutes, stirring every 15 minutes.
7. Remove large clumps and let it cool to room temperature.
8. Enjoy!

Yields: 18 servings - 2/3 cup servings
Cal: 116.7 | P: 0.7g | C: 27.7 g | F: 2.8 g

Carrot Pumpkin Bars

Ingredients
2 teaspoons baking powder
1 teaspoon baking soda
2 cups flour
1 ¼ teaspoon pumpkin pie spice
½ cup brown sugar
1 cup sugar
1/3 cup light margarine/butter – softened
2 large egg whites (+) 2 large whole eggs
1 can (15 ounces) pumpkin pie filling
1 cup finely shredded carrots

For the Topping:
¼ cup sugar
4 ounces softened cream cheese
1 tablespoon skim milk

Instructions
1. Program the oven setting to 350°F.
2. Lightly grease a rectangular dish/jellyroll pan
3. Mix the baking powder, baking soda, pumpkin spice, and sugar.
4. In a large mixing dish, whisk the brown sugar, white sugar, and butter until it crumbles. Blend in the pie mix,

carrots, and all eggs along with the flour mixture. Spread into the pan.

5. For the cream cheese topping; blend the sugar, milk, and cream cheese. Drop by the teaspoonful into the batter and swirl with a knife.
6. Bake 25-30 minutes. Cool in the pan and cut into the squares

Yields: 24 servings
Cal: 131.6 | P: 2.8 g | C: 28.5 g | F: 1.7 g

Chocolate Brownie

Ingredients
1 tablespoon each of:
- Whole wheat flour
- Sugar (no substitutes)
- Unsweetened cocoa
- Low-fat yogurt (+) more if needed to blend

1 pinch of:
- Baking soda
- Salt

Instructions
1. Combine the fixings in a mug.
2. Pop it into the microwave for one minute.

Yields: One serving
Cal: 94.5 | P: 2.6 g | C: 22.1 g | F: 1.1 g

Cinnamon Almond Raisins Snack

Ingredients
1 teaspoon cinnamon
1 cup of each:
- Raisins
- Almonds

Instructions

1. Rinse the almonds and raisins in water.
2. Add them to a food processor with the cinnamon.
3. Balls will form when mixed.
4. Divide them into 12 balls and enjoy.

Yields: Six servings (2 balls per serving)
Cal: 219.6 | P: 5.9 g | C: 27.2g | F: 11.8g

Granola and Nut Bars

Ingredients
2 cups rolled oats
1 cup quick-cooking oats
1/8 teaspoon salt
½ teaspoon cinnamon
¼ cup raw almonds
1 – 1 ½ - tablespoons canola/olive oil
¼ cup each:
  - Honey
  - Vanilla-flavored almond milk
  - Shredded coconut
1/3 cup pure maple syrup
Non-stick cooking spray

Instructions

1. Program the toaster oven/oven to 350°F.
2. Process the rolled oats in a blender or food processor until they are flour-like. Mix the oat flour with everything dry except for the coconut.
3. Add the wet components and stir until well mixed.
4. Spray a baking dish with the mixture, pressing it down with a spatula, and add the coconut as the top layer.
5. Slice the sheet into 12 bars and bake 15 to 20 minutes.
6. Let the treats chill and slice again for storage.

Yields: 12 servings
Cal: 220.4 | P: 6.9 g | C: 39.6 g | F: 5.4 g

Peanut Butter Chocolate Protein Bars – No-Bake

Ingredients
3 tablespoons honey
1 cup uncooked oats
1 cup 'natural' peanut butter
1 ½ cups chocolate whey protein powder
2 –5 tablespoons water
1 tablespoon unsweetened cocoa –*optional*

Instructions
1. In a microwavable dish, add and cook the honey and peanut butter for 30 seconds.
2. Blend in the remainder of the fixings and mix together.
3. Press the mixture hard into a square dish, and let it set in the fridge for 20 minutes.

Yields: 12 servings
Cal: 221 | P: 15.5 g | C: 12.8 g | F: 11.1g

Peanut Butter Cookies (No-Bake & Gluten-free)

Ingredients
1 large egg
1 cup natural peanut butter
1 cup sugar

Instructions
1. Set the oven temperature to 375°F.
2. Combine the fixings, and scoop out the dough into one-inch balls.

3. Arrange on a cookie sheet two inches apart and flatten with a fork.
4. Cook nine minutes, remove and let cool a few minutes on the baking sheet.

Note: As they cool, they will become firm.

Yields: 36 cookies/servings
Cal: 67.9 | P: 1.7g | C: 6.9 g | F: 3.7 g

Drinks

Ginger Pomegranate Spritzer

Ingredients
1 bottle (12 ounces) non-alcoholic ginger beer
16 ounces pomegranate juice
Juice of 2 limes

Instructions
1. Mix all of the ingredients
2. Serve in chilled win goblets for a special treat!

Yields: Four servings
Cal: 116.0 | P: 0.1 g | C: 29.5 g | F: 0 g

Iced Coffee

Ingredients
1 tablespoon each:
- Instant coffee
- Chocolate instant breakfast (Carnation)

5 ounces cold water
2 ounces each:
- Hot water
- Fat-free milk

2-3 packs Splenda
1 tablespoon coffee creamer – Hazelnut
Ice cubes

Instructions
1. Blend the coffee, breakfast mix, and hot water in a 16 ounce glass.
2. Add the milk, cold water, and creamer.
3. Stir and top it off with the ice.

Yields: One serving
Cal: 75.7 | P: 2.9 g | C: 15.3 g | F: 0.1 g

Lemonade

Ingredients
5 cups water
1 cup fresh lemon juice
½ cup/24 packets Splenda
Ice cubes
Optional:
- Raspberries
- Mint sprigs
- Lemon slices

Instructions
1. Combine all of the ingredients into a large pitcher.
2. Serve over ice and garnish as desired.

Yields: Eight servings
Cal: 7.6 | P: 0.1 g | C: 6.2 g | F: 0 g

Frosty Peach Shake

Ingredients
½ cup each:
- Frozen strawberries
- Skim milk

1 cup ach:
- Non-fat peach yogurt
- Frozen/canned peaches

Instructions
1. Blend all of these tasty ingredients in the blender until creamy smooth!

Yields: Two servings
Cal: 234.0 | P: 7.7 g | C: 49.1 g | F: 2.2 g

Pumpkin Protein Shake

Ingredients
1/3 cup each:
  2% evaporated milk
  Canned pumpkin puree
1 cup vanilla flavored soy milk
2 Splenda packets
1 scoop vanilla protein powder
To Taste: Nutmeg and cinnamon
6 ice cubes

Instructions
1. Add the ice along with the wet and dry ingredients to the blender.
2. Blend until you reach the desired consistency.
3. Pour into your glass and go!

Yields: One serving
Cal: 263.7 | P: 27.6 g | C: 28.2 g | F: 5.5 g

Strawberry Cheesecake Shake

Ingredients
2 cups frozen – unsweetened strawberries
4 – 8 packages Splenda/your choice brand
½ cup each:
- Low-fat 1% cottage cheese
- 1% milk

Optional: ½ teaspoon almond/vanilla extract

Instructions
1. Blend the cottage cheese, milk, extract, and sweetener in the blender (about 30 seconds).
2. Add the frozen berries once the cheese mixture is smooth.

Yields: Two servings or one for a filling meal
Cal: 236.3 | P: 19.4 g | C: 36.4 g | F: 2.7 g

Conclusion

Thank for making it through to the end of the *Bariatric Cookbook: Delicious Recipes for Your Gastric Sleeve Recovery.* Let's hope it was informative and provided you with all of the tools you need to achieve your goals, whatever they may be.

The next step is to head out to the supermarket and get some of the ingredients needed to get you started with your new way of life. You have made two huge steps towards a better way of living. Now, you can make the dream a reality with these new ways to enjoy food that you never imagined could be so healthy.

Finally, if you found this book useful in any way, a review on Amazon is always appreciated!

Index

Chapter 1: Breakfast

Muffins

Oats

Pancakes

Cold Breakfast Treats

- Chocolate Covered Strawberries Smoothie
- Going Green Smoothie
- Mixed Berry Smoothie
- Peanut Butter Banana Smoothie
- Pumpkin Smoothie
- Strawberry Banana Smoothie
- Yogurt Breakfast Popsicles

Chapter 2: Lunch: Salads and Pasta Dishes

Salads

- Caprese Salad
- California Roll in a Bowl
- Caramel Apple Salad
- Chickpea and Feta Salad
- Coleslaw
- Cucumber and Onion Salad with Vinegar
- Egg Salad
- Grape Salad
- Israeli Salad
- Sunshine Fruit Salad

Pasta Dishes

- Skillet Lasagna
- Mediterranean Salmon with Pasta
- Shrimp Pasta

Chapter 3: Lunch: Soups Stews and Sandwiches

Soups and Stews

- Cabbage Vegetable Soup
- Chicken Tortilla Soup – Slow Cooker
- Fifteen Minute Chili
- 5 Ingredient Soup
- French Onion Soup
- Potato Soup – Slow Cooker
- **Tomato Soup**

Sandwiches

- BBQ Steak/Chicken Wrap
- Buffalo Chicken Sandwich
- Cheesy Salsa Dog
- Crab Melt
- Hawaiian Turkey Burger
- Ranch Cheddar Turkey Burgers
- Vegetarian Philly Cheese steak Sandwich

Chapter 4: Dinner Dishes

Chicken
- Chicken Broccoli and Tomato Stir Fry
- Chicken and Broccoli Casserole

Beef
- Bavarian Beef
- BBQ Steak/Chicken Wrap

- DC Sloppy Jo
- Ginger Beef
- Ground Beef Casserole – Keema
- Ground Beef and Potato Casserole
- Mushroom and Beef - Slow Cooker
- Slimmer Beef Stroganoff - Stir Fry

Chicken and Turkey

- Baked Chicken and Vegetables
- Brown Sugar Garlic Chicken
- Chicken Creole
- Chicken Enchiladas and Sour Cream
- Chicken Tetrazzini
- Cola Chicken
- Creamy Italian Chicken – Slow Cooker

Fish

- BBQ Roasted Salmon
- Breaded Cod Fillet
- Broiled Tilapia Parmesan
- Mock Crab Cakes
- Oven-Fried Tilapia
- Salmon – Quick and Easy
- Salmon Patties

Pork

- Asian Pork Tenderloin
- BBQ Pulled Pork Roast – Slow Cooker
- Grilled Honey Garlic Pork Chops
- Mustard Brown Sugar Pork Chops

Chapter 5: Vegetarian Dishes

- Black Bean and Rice Casserole
- Broccoli Casserole
- Eggplant Pesto Mini Pizza
- Quinoa and Black Bean Casserole
- Vegetable Curry – Slow Cooker
- Vegetarian Chili
- Vegetarian Lentil Loaf
- Veggie Frittata

Chapter 6: Snacks, Desserts, and Drinks

Snacks

- Cheese Quesadilla
- Chili Popcorn
- Hummus
- Roasted Kale Chips

Desserts - Sweet Snacks

- Banana Nut Granola
- Caramel Popcorn
- Carrot Pumpkin Bars
- Chocolate Brownie
- Cinnamon Almond Raisins Snack
- Granola and Nut Bars
- Peanut Butter Chocolate Protein Bars – No-Bake
- Peanut Butter Cookies (No-Bake & Gluten-free)

Drinks

- Ginger Pomegranate Spritzer
- Lemonade
- Frosty Peach Shake
- Pumpkin Protein Shake
- Strawberry Cheesecake Shake